CELEBRATE YOUR
FEELINGS

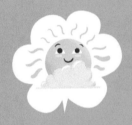

CELEBRATE YOUR
FEELINGS

THE POSITIVE MINDSET
PUBERTY BOOK FOR GIRLS

BY LAUREN RIVERS, MS

Illustrated by CAIT BRENNAN

ROCKRIDGE
PRESS

For general information on our other products and services or to obtain technical support, please contact our Customer Care Department within the United States at (866) 744-2665, or outside the United States at (510) 253-0500.

Rockridge Press publishes its books in a variety of electronic and print formats. Some content that appears in print may not be available in electronic books, and vice versa.

TRADEMARKS: Rockridge Press and the Rockridge Press logo are trademarks or registered trademarks of Callisto Media Inc. and/or its affiliates, in the United States and other countries, and may not be used without written permission. All other trademarks are the property of their respective owners. Rockridge Press is not associated with any product or vendor mentioned in this book.

Interior and Cover Designer: Tricia Jang
Art Producer: Hannah Dickerson
Editor: Eun H. Jeong
Production Editor: Emily Sheehan
Illustrations © Cait Brennan
Decorative patterns courtesy of Shutterstock
Author photo courtesy of Clark Douglas
ISBN: Print 978-1-64739-289-5 | eBook 978-1-64739-290-1
R0

TO MY MOM,
who, due to her unconditional
support, constant listening ear, and
kind spirit, has taught me more about
what it takes to be a counselor than
any course or textbook.

TO MYRA,
for loving us as your own.

AND TO ANY GIRL
wondering whether things gets better—
they most certainly do.

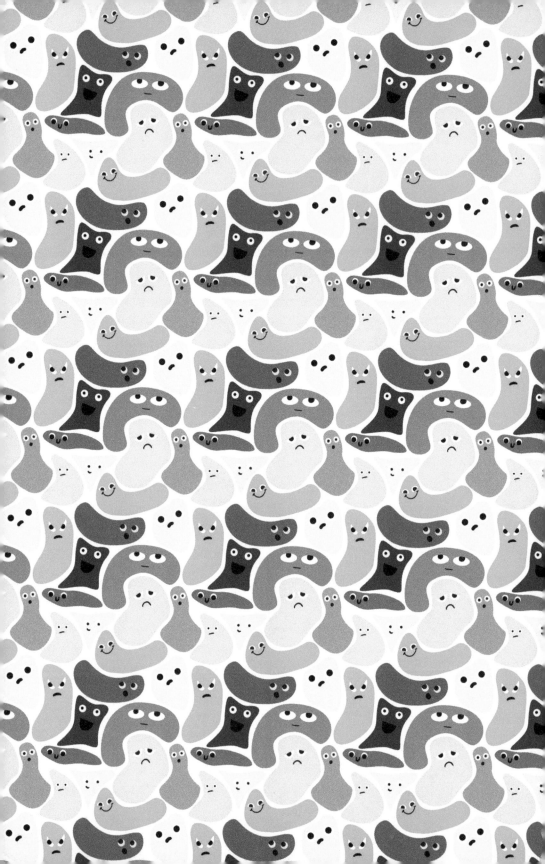

CONTENTS

Dear Reader,

You may not realize it, but every day you are changing and growing. When you were younger, you might have felt scared when someone yelled, but maybe now you feel angry. Or maybe you once loved to sing in front of people, but now you feel shy or want to run and hide from attention. These new feelings can leave you confused or with a lot of questions. I remember being VERY confused!

When I was your age, I experienced all kinds of emotions. Sometimes it felt like a roller coaster as my feelings soared from sad to joyful to angry—sometimes all in a single day. (Can you relate to this?) During puberty, I got a lot of advice from parents and teachers on how my body was changing, but nobody talked to me about all the changes I was experiencing inside of me. I wasn't sure if what I was going through was normal. I was nervous, but also curious.

My curiosity continued to grow, and I decided to study clinical mental health counseling at Johns Hopkins University and to work in elementary schools, offices, and hospitals in Baltimore, Maryland, and Northern Virginia. And now my job is to help adolescents like you navigate through these social and emotional changes. I love my job, and I've met some amazing young girls. As I help them, I learn so much from them, too. It's been a lot of fun. Now, I'm excited to take all that I've learned and put it in the book you're holding!

This book will help you feel excited for these amazing changes and will teach you super-helpful skills to manage your emotions, relationships, thoughts, and moods. By the end of this book, I believe you will know yourself and appreciate yourself better. You'll also have what it takes to connect with others as a strong, smart, and confident person.

I look forward to joining you on this new adventure!

Yours truly,
Lauren Rivers

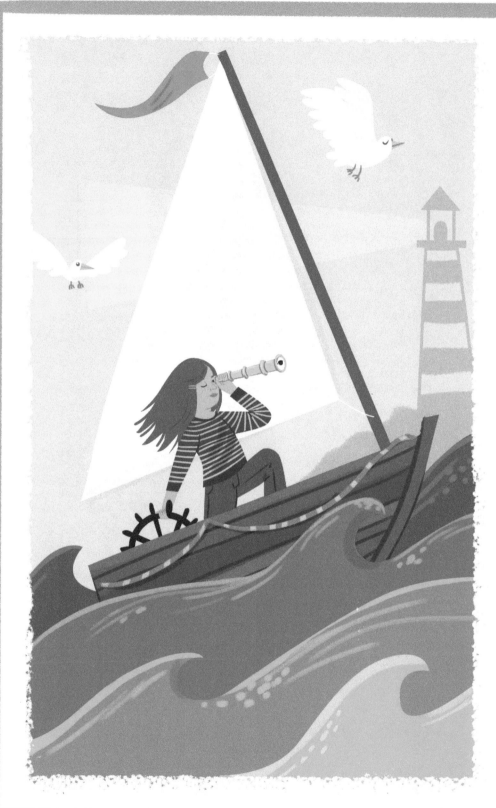

MY CHANGING EMOTIONS

· ·

You are unique. You are special. You are awesome. Uncertainty about your feelings might keep you from seeing that, and that's normal! The more you understand your feelings and emotions, the less confused you will feel as you grow and change. You may not realize it, but you already have everything you need inside you to handle these changes. But certain tools and tricks can make it much easier— and that's where this book comes in.

Have you ever burst into tears or stomped your feet when someone made you angry? Did you ever feel like you were about to cry in class and tried your hardest to stop yourself? Your feelings might be different from those of a family member, best friend, or favorite teacher. That's okay! There's no limit to how many emotions you can feel, and there's no right or wrong way to have them, either. Have you ever wondered why you cover your eyes or jump during the scary part of a movie? Well, your feelings affect how your body reacts! Pretty neat stuff, huh? But our feelings don't just affect our body—they also impact the way we see ourselves, treat our friends, and experience the world around us.

WHAT AM I FEELING?

Think of yourself as the captain of your emotions, on a boat in a big, beautiful sea of growth and change. Your feelings are a lot like waves. Sometimes feelings can be huge, choppy, scary waves. Sometimes you're happy because the waves are small and smooth—of course, this is when it's easier to navigate the boat.

Emotions and feelings are words that help describe how we feel on the inside. We have emotions and feelings all day long. Some emotions are nice and can make us feel warm and fuzzy, like excitement. Others, like anger, are tougher, and we may try to ignore them. Emotions are our response, or our reaction, to things that happen to us. Our emotions create feelings, and our feelings cause our moods to change. Your mood might change from happy in the morning to sad in the afternoon and then back to happy before bedtime. You might tell a friend, "I just don't feel like myself today," after fighting with a sibling. Negative emotions might keep you from feeling like your normal, happy self for a little bit. It might not always seem like it, but if you know what to do, you can handle your changing moods, no matter the size of the waves.

MY FEELINGS

Have you ever known a friend or classmate who got a new puppy? Maybe you were jealous at first but then felt happy for them. We can have so many different feelings in a short span of time, but the better you become at identifying your feelings, the more prepared you will be to navigate your boat! Circle any feelings you've had today or in the past few days:

Confident	Annoyed	Relaxed
Serious	Stressed	Brave
Frustrated	Respectful	Moody
Kind	Calm	Silly
Joyful	Jealous	Anxious
Sad	Happy	Grumpy
Loving	Curious	Embarrassed
Excited	Impulsive	Fearful
Confused	Angry	Proud
Hopeful	Strong	Worried

Expressing Emotions

It's important to feel like you can be yourself, even when you're having strong emotions. If you didn't get to wear your favorite outfit for picture day, you might feel disappointed, and your mood may shift from happy to sad. You may be less talkative when you're upset or want to be left alone. When this happens, your friends may comment or ask what's wrong. This means that you've expressed yourself in a way that tells others a story about how you feel. Emotional expression is the way you choose to show your feelings. There is no wrong or right way to do this, but some ways of expressing your emotions are healthier than others.

Brain Talk

There are five main parts of the brain that help shape our emotions and actions. Let's call them the brain's VIPs (Very Important Parts). Four of the VIPs are the **amygdala**, **hippocampus**, **thalamus**, and **hypothalamus**. They help shape the way we act and feel, and they make up our **limbic system**, the fifth VIP. The limbic system is an area of the brain that manages most of our emotions, feelings, and moods. Although these VIPs have different responsibilities, they come together to do one important job: keep us safe, alert, and healthy. You know when your teacher asks you to sit quietly throughout the day so class will run smoothly? These VIPs kind of do the same for your brain.

Amygdala (uh-mig-duh-luh) This is a small but mighty part of your brain. Think of the amygdala as the engine of your boat. It manages many of your emotions—especially fear. Fear is a helpful emotion that keeps us safe from harm. If your amygdala senses harm, your body will produce hormones to help keep you safe. You may notice sweaty hands or a faster heartbeat. This "fight, flight, or freeze" response can help you protect yourself in dangerous situations.

Hypothalamus (hy-poh-thal-uh-mus) Have you ever felt grumpy at school because you couldn't sleep the night before? This brain structure really wants you to get enough sleep so you're in a good mood the next day. The hypothalamus helps create a sleep pattern

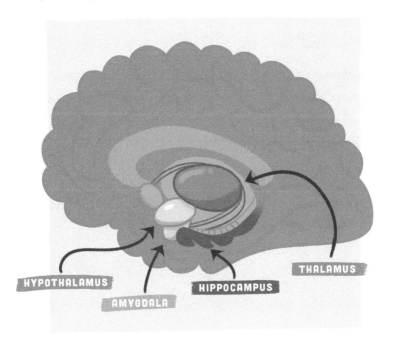

that your body is used to. It also helps you notice when you're hungry, thirsty, too hot, or too cold. All of these things can change your mood!

Hippocampus (hip-poh-camp-us) This one sounds like an African animal, but it's a super-cool part of your brain! Have you ever driven by a friend's old house after they moved and instantly felt sad? The hippocampus helps your brain with memory by connecting it with an emotion and sometimes even a smell. Maybe your younger brother is starting kindergarten in your old classroom, and the smell of that room brings back memories from when you were his age. This is your hippocampus at work. Speaking of the classroom, this part of the brain helps you remember what you've read and learned. If you remember some things from this book, you can thank your hippocampus!

Thalamus (thal-uh-mus) This is the great emotional messenger of our brain. Once your amygdala experiences an emotion, the thalamus sends signals through your brain to help you understand it. Think of it as a mailroom that receives a ton of important letters telling us how to feel and respond to what's going on around us.

Levels of Feelings

All our feelings come from basic or "primary" emotions. The six primary emotions are happiness, sadness, anger, fear, disgust, and surprise. These primary emotions are what you notice first, right after something has happened. Then you might start to feel "secondary" emotions. If you get a bad grade on a test, your primary emotion might be sadness and your secondary might be worry, when you think about what your parents will say.

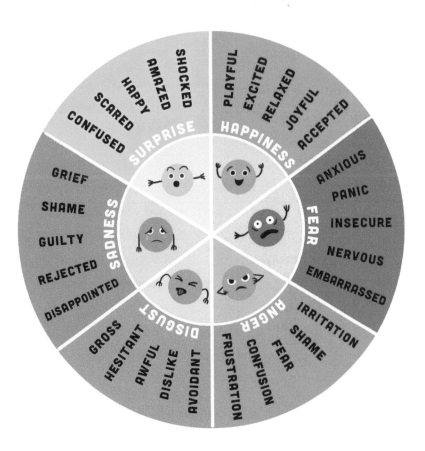

Helpful Hormones

Hormones are chemicals that our brain sends to different parts of our body so change and growth can happen. Hormones can also help you feel ready to run when you're scared, happy when you hug your parent, proud of yourself when you do well at school, or embarrassed when someone makes fun of you. Let's explore:

Oxytocin (oxy-tos-in) Scientists call this the love hormone because it helps us feel and express love. This hormone helps us feel safe, secure, and less anxious. When you hug your best friend, your body releases oxytocin. This explains why it feels so good to love and be loved in return!

Serotonin and dopamine (ser-uh-ton-in), (doh-puh-meen) These are our happy hormones. Have you ever made an A on a test and felt proud of yourself? Well, this is because your hard work paid off and your body released dopamine to reward you. The more accomplished you feel, the more dopamine your brain is making. Serotonin is what your body releases when you play outside or run around the gym. The more you exercise your body, the more serotonin your body makes and the better you feel. This is why exercise is good for your mood. If you don't have enough dopamine or serotonin, you may feel moody or sad or have trouble paying attention.

Adrenaline and cortisol (uh-dren-ah-lin), (cor-ti-sol)

Think of these hormones as your defenders. Remember the "fight, flight, or freeze" response we talked about? Adrenaline and cortisol help keep you safe from harm by preparing your body to run, fight back, or freeze in place. These hormones can be helpful or harmful. If you're on a road trip with your family and another car almost hits you, these hormones will help your parent react fast so everyone in the car can stay safe. But these hormones can be harmful when your body thinks it's in trouble when it's not. Like if your body tells you you're in danger because you failed a quiz at school, it will make these hormones even though they aren't very helpful in that situation. It's a wonderful thing that your body is trying to keep you safe from harm, but it's important to know when you are or aren't in actual danger. The next section will show you some of the ways you can handle your emotions in these types of situations.

MY EMOTIONAL SCORE

How well do you understand emotions? Take this quiz to find out! Read the statement, and then decide how well it describes you.

1. When I am feeling angry or frustrated, I know that these are normal emotions that will go away soon.

   a. Yes, most of the time
   b. Sometimes
   c. No, not usually

2. I show my friends I care about them by asking them how they're feeling.

   a. Yes, most of the time
   b. Sometimes
   c. No, not usually

3. I know that my mood can affect others around me and that their mood can affect me, too.

   a. Yes, most of the time
   b. Sometimes
   c. No, not usually

4. I try to be kind and cheerful to my friends, even when I am feeling grumpy or sad.

   a. Yes, most of the time

b. Sometimes

c. No, not usually

5. When I feel sad or think I might cry, I talk to a trusted grown-up or friend instead of keeping it bottled up inside.

a. Yes, most of the time

b. Sometimes

c. No, not usually

6. I'm a good listener when my friends are having a bad day, because I know what it's like to have a bad day, too.

a. Yes, most of the time

b. Sometimes

c. No, not usually

7. I know that emotions are a normal part of being human and everyone feels and expresses them differently.

a. Yes, most of the time

b. Sometimes

c. No, not really

8. When I am confused about my feelings, I talk about them with a trusted grown-up.

a. Yes, most of the time

b. Sometimes

c. No, not usually

Give yourself 3 points for every a, 2 points for every b, and 1 point for every c.

Did you score an 18 or above? Woohoo! You're off to a great start navigating your changing feelings and emotions. Keep reading this book to learn even more about yourself.

If you scored under 18, don't worry! We're all learning together, and you should feel proud of what you already know. Congratulate yourself for answering honestly, and keep reading for lots of advice and activities that will help you learn so much more.

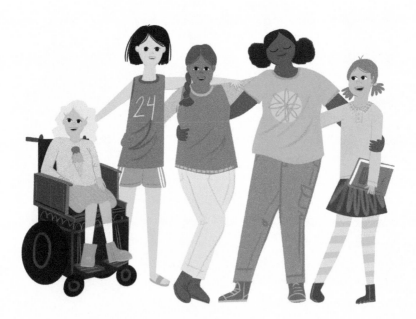

HOW CAN I FEEL BETTER?

We all have emotions—lots of them. But it's important to know how to deal with them in a way that leaves you feeling better, not worse. There are no right or wrong emotions to have, but there are some not-so-nice ways of expressing yourself, such as fighting or yelling. I'm going to share some tips and tricks for handling your emotions. They can help you feel better when you feel bad and can help you express yourself in the healthiest way. When you're able to express yourself in a calmer or kinder manner, your friendships and relationships with others are better, too. Let's talk about some of these techniques:

Breathe deeply.

Thankfully, breathing is so automatic that we never have to think about doing it! Sometimes, though, it can be helpful to notice your breaths and prac-tice breathing deeply and slowly. Deep breathing lowers your feelings of anx-iety and can make you feel 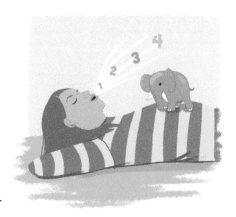 calm and even sleepy. There are a couple of fun ways to practice deep breathing:

Take a big, deep breath in for four seconds, hold it for another four seconds, and then slowly exhale for another four seconds. Repeat this a few times until you feel calm.

Place your favorite stuffed animal or blanket on your tummy and watch it go up and down as you take big, deep breaths in and out.

Relax those muscles.

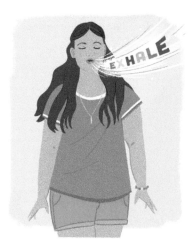

When we feel stressed out, our brain sends a message to the body to prepare for danger. This causes our muscles to feel tense. If this happens a lot, it can cause pain throughout your body, such as headaches or sore shoulders. To relax your tight muscles, try this:

Take a big breath in, and squeeze those muscles until they feel tight or tense. Then relax and slowly let go of the pressure, breathing out as you go. For example, try putting both of your fists into a tight ball and holding it for a few seconds before letting go slowly. When you let go, breathe out slowly and count to 10. It's helpful to relax your shoulders and jaw as you release, too.

Exercise it out.

Exercise is great for your mind *and* body. Here's how to get some happy hormones going inside you:

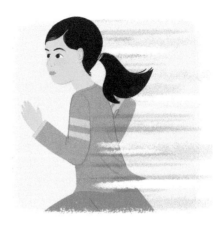

Next time you're feeling angry or sluggish, or just looking for something to do, turn to your favorite exercise: run, dance, bike, whatever! Ask a parent to take you to dance, karate, or swim practice for an extra dose of these hormones. Grab a friend or sibling and jump rope, walk, toss a ball, or hula-hoop—it all counts.

Sleep tight.

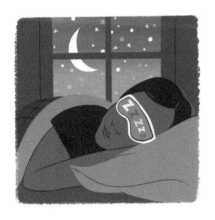

Did you know your body does important work while you sleep? If you sleep less than nine hours, your body probably didn't get to do all its work, so you may feel grumpy or sleepy. You may feel too tired in class to answer questions, which could leave you feeling disappointed in yourself. Here are a few ways to make sure you're getting good sleep at night:

- ◆ Go to bed around the same time each night.
- ◆ Avoid sugary drinks before bed.
- ◆ Try not to eat dinner right before bed.
- ◆ Turn off electronics an hour before bedtime.
- ◆ Read a book or listen to calming music or sounds.

Find your safe space.

Close your eyes and let your imagination take over! I want you to imagine and describe your happiest or safest place. This can be a real place you've been, or you can make it up and decorate it how you want. Be sure to include:

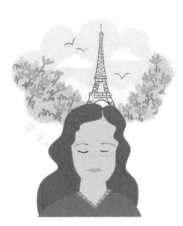

- ◆ The sights, including the color of the walls or sky
- ◆ The smells
- ◆ The temperature
- ◆ The sounds
- ◆ What you're wearing
- ◆ Who is or isn't there

Be as detailed and creative as you want—you may even want to imagine what superpowers you have!

Want to relax even more? Do this activity along with deep breathing.

MY FAVORITE THINGS

Good memories can always make us smile. Did you know that one way to handle difficult emotions is to look back on your favorite memories? These memories might be from when you laughed so hard with a friend that you both couldn't talk or a favorite vacation. Scrapbooking is a fun way to put all those memories in one special place.

To get started, visit your nearest crafts store or "go shopping" in your house with materials you already own. You may want to use scrapbook or construction paper, markers, pens, colored pencils, stickers, stamps, favorite photos you are allowed to cut and glue, safe scissors, glue, stencils, or anything else that makes you happy.

Start by setting aside a page for each of your favorite memories. Now get creative and fill the scrapbook with your most special memories. You can turn to it whenever you're feeling down.

Practice mindfulness.

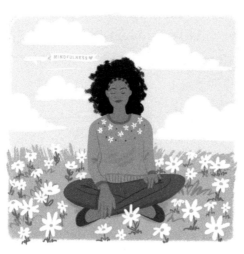

Do you ever feel that your thoughts and feelings are like a loud storm in your head? Sometimes you may wish you could quiet that storm. You can, and here's how:

Try to imagine your thoughts or feelings as clouds passing by in the sky. When you watch the clouds, you simply notice and appreciate them for what they are. You can do this with your thoughts, too! Try "sitting with them," imagining them as clouds passing by or labeling them with feeling words.

For example, you could say to yourself, "I know I am feeling sadness. I am going to sit with it until it goes by on its own because I know it will." Mindfulness doesn't make your thoughts or feelings go away, but it helps you accept them and enjoy the present moment, instead of worrying about the past or the future.

Here's another mindfulness trick: Slowly draw your name in fun letters on a piece of paper. Pay attention to each stroke of the marker, noticing the shapes you're creating, while also paying attention to your thoughts and feelings as you go along.

Find ways to practice self-care.

Self-care is exactly what it sounds like—taking care of yourself! Here's a self-care exercise that can help you feel good about yourself:

Start by making two lists. Create one list with some of your favorite activities. It could be taking a bath, going to the movies, or eating pizza. Make a second list with some activities that you don't always want to do but know you'd feel proud of afterward, like doing a chore or getting started on a school project.

Notice how both lists help you take care of yourself—sometimes in a fun way, other times in a way that will help your future self. Self-care sets you up to feel good tomorrow, next week, and next year.

Now combine each list and do one or a few self-care activities every day. Mix it up—do things from both lists. Self-care activities, whether practicing your favorite sport or raking the leaves in the yard, help you feel better because you are having fun and relaxing while still taking care of your needs and responsibilities.

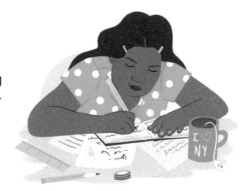

Use good body language.

Body language is the way we hold our shoulders, the volume of our voice, the way we move our hands, and our eye contact and facial expressions. It tells others a lot about us and how we're feeling. Do you slump your shoul- 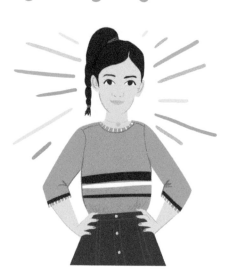 ders when someone picks on you? Do you sit up straight and shoot up your hand when you know an answer? As you can see, body language can be positive or negative, but positive body language makes us feel better and more confident! Here are two ways to help you become aware of body language and use it to change how you feel:

Stand in front of a mirror. Practice how you might appear if you were scared, or embarrassed, or proud. Notice how your face and posture and body show your feelings. How can you change these to be more positive?

Practice confident body language. Try standing up straight, speaking up clearly, or doing a superhero pose in front of the mirror. And when you feel negative body language coming on, use these tricks to stand proud!

Talk it out.

Feelings can be overwhelming! Talking to a friend, family member, or trusted grown-up is a great way to make sense of your feelings. When you are upset, or even experiencing several different emotions, you might feel confused and stressed.

Talking to someone you trust can help you figure out why you're feeling those emotions. More importantly, talking things through can make you feel better and not so alone.

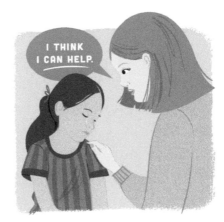

The next time you feel stressed, seek out a trusted grown-up to talk to. You may not want to immediately talk about what's bothering you, and that's okay. Just spending time with someone who cares about you can help you feel better and more relaxed, and you may soon feel comfortable enough to open up to them.

Who Is a "Trusted Grown-up"?

Talking to your friends about your feelings is okay and can be helpful at times, but a trusted grown-up might be able to help more because they have already experienced many of the same feelings you're having, and they can give you advice and support. A trusted grown-up is someone you feel comfortable and safe around. They want you to feel happy and would never hurt you physically or emotionally. They will not ask you to keep secrets from other adults or to do or say anything you aren't comfortable with. This might be a parent, school counselor, teacher, coach, or grandparent.

Not everyone is a trusted grown-up. Always remember, if you get a weird gut feeling when talking to someone, pay attention to this feeling, because this person might not be what you consider a trusted grown-up.

When you want to talk to a trusted grown-up, start by telling them how you're feeling. For example, you can say, "I'm sad that my friends left me out, and I want to talk about it when you have time."

The more you practice turning to a trusted grown-up in your life, the more confident you'll become talking about your feelings!

I KNOW WHAT TO DO!

You just learned all kinds of tricks for handling your emotions—now see if you can connect each situation below with a good trick to deal with it. Happy matching!

Feeling jealous of the new girl

Find a safe space

Feeling angry at your best friend for spending more time with another friend

Do some deep breathing

Feeling anxious in the car or on a road trip with your family

Exercise mindfulness

Feeling embarrassed after missing the ball during a softball game

Practice self-care

Feeling proud after getting a good grade on your math quiz

Change your body language

Feeling disappointed that your mom or dad couldn't chaperone the field trip

Exercise

Feeling sad or unmotivated to do your favorite things

Talk it out

Did you find good tricks for each situation? Everyone is different, and there is no wrong answer. Each of these tricks can be helpful for any situation.

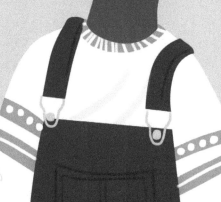

MY CHANGING MIND

• •

Now you know that every single day, you're growing and changing. Hopefully, you're also realizing you can think harder, juggle more responsibilities, and be yourself with your friends and family. Would you have thought five years ago that one day you'd be able to make your own lunch, play a sport, get good grades, and be a good friend, all at the same time? That's the exciting part of growth and change. Some changes you go through can be unexpected, but everyone goes through them, and guess what? There is no right or wrong way to feel. As these changes happen, if you can learn to manage your emotions in a positive way, it will leave you feeling empowered—like you can handle anything!

A POSITIVE MINDSET

All of these changing emotions can be confusing! You may notice that your emotions feel stronger when you're hungry or tired, or when you get bad news. It's true that our emotions affect how we feel, think, and act, but it's important to know that they don't make us who we are. We are separate from our emotions, just like we are separate from our mistakes. You can make a mistake and still be a good person, just like you can feel sad but still be your happy, joyful self at the end of the day. The best way to do this is to notice your changing emotions, deal with them, but remain the awesome person you are.

Even if you are a positive person, you may experience a negative emotion or have a bad day, and it might feel like you're never going to get back to that happy, bubbly personality of yours. Thankfully, this isn't true! Positive and negative emotions come and go, but it's how you act when you feel them that matters.

Positive emotions can cause positive actions, while negative emotions can cause negative actions. Sometimes, when we're experiencing a tough emotion, we accidentally do things that make us feel worse, like yell at someone we care about. In between this feeling and action, there is usually a thought. This thought is your inner voice! Your inner voice helps you decide if you're going to make a healthy decision, like to talk calmly, or an unhealthy one, like to yell.

Let's think of your negative and positive thoughts as colors, like **RED** and **GREEN**.

A negative inner voice, or red thought, might sound like, "No one asked me to join their group in art today. It's probably because I'm bad at painting. I'm just going to quit trying." A positive inner voice, or green thought, might sound like, "I was able to paint alone today, and I paint really well when I'm not distracted. I am proud of myself, but tomorrow I'd like to ask my friends if they want to work together."

Your inner voice is powerful, and it might feel impossible to stop the red thoughts, but with a little practice, you can change your negative mindset by turning your red thoughts into green ones. Here's how:

1. Notice the negative thought.
2. Challenge yourself to find something good in the situation.
3. Reword the thought so it focuses on the good things instead of the bad.

Here are some examples of turning red thoughts into green ones:

RED THOUGHT: My best friend didn't sit next to me at lunch today. She must not like me anymore.

GREEN THOUGHT: My best friend chose to sit next to a new friend today, and I know it has nothing to do with how she feels about me. I'm proud of her because I know that's hard. There will be a day when I do that, too. I'd like to be the kind of friend who is accepting of my friends' decisions.

RED THOUGHT: I go to a separate classroom to get more help with reading. I must not be as smart as my classmates.

GREEN THOUGHT: I get the chance to go to a new classroom and have fun one-on-one time with my reading teacher. There are no distractions in there, and I've already learned a ton.

Another helpful way of quieting your red thoughts would be to label them and say, "Hey, I know this is a red thought, and my red thoughts usually aren't true. Hmm, let me think of a green thought on that subject!"

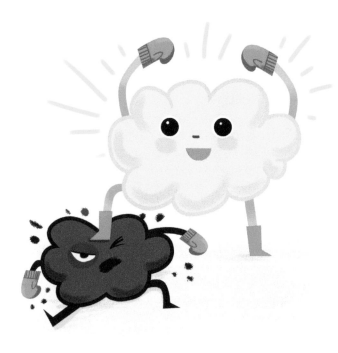

POSITIVE SELF-TALK

Complete a green thought by thinking about the positive in the situation instead of the negative.

RED: Charlie made fun of me for not spending the night away from home yet. She probably thinks I'm a baby.

GREEN: _____

_____

_____

RED: I heard my parents arguing last night about me and my brother. Is it our fault that they fight?

GREEN: _____

_____

_____

RED: I became angry at my teammate during soccer practice because she didn't do what she was supposed to. She probably won't speak to me now.

GREEN: _____

_____

_____

Fill in your own red and green thoughts for the last three:

RED: _____

_____

_____

GREEN: _____

_____

_____

RED: _____

_____

_____

GREEN: _____

_____

_____

RED: _____

_____

_____

GREEN: _____

_____

_____

FROM SELF-CONSCIOUS TO CONFIDENT

Do you ever feel like your classmates are watching everything you say and do? Maybe you tried to wear your clothes from last year and realized you've grown out of them. These are self-conscious thoughts and feelings, and they're super common in kids your age. Feeling self-conscious simply means you're very aware of yourself, and that is not always a bad thing. It can help you be thoughtful about your words and actions. You should give yourself a high-five for being so in tune with yourself! But too much self-consciousness can be negative and make you feel like you're not good enough.

Confidence is when you trust yourself and feel proud of your skills and who you are. Confidence can take time to grow, because it comes from trying new things, facing your fears, and getting lots of practice. Maybe you remember feeling proud of yourself after scoring a goal at your soccer game. This helped build your confidence because it showed you what you're capable of.

But you don't always have to be "good" at things to feel confident. If you know you worked hard, practiced, and tried your best, your confidence is also growing, and that's exciting. You can even grow your confidence by loving and accepting yourself for who you are and not worrying about what others think of you.

Want to trade self-consciousness for confidence? Try these tips:

+ If you're feeling self-conscious about your looks, try standing in front of the mirror in a strong, proud pose and say three things you love about yourself out loud. They can be about anything! Just focus on being you and not on what you think others think of you.

+ If you're feeling self-conscious about participating in an activity or exercising in PE, try practicing some of these exercises at home with family or friends, such as going for a run. Sometimes, practicing things that you're worried about will help give you the confidence to do them later.

Once you've done these activities, try writing what you liked about them in a journal so you can look back and feel proud of yourself for your progress.

Media Messages

Have you ever looked in the mirror and wished you looked different in some way? Body image is the way we view ourselves and feel about our body. We are so lucky to have the bodies that we do, no matter the shape, size, or ability, but sometimes it's easy to forget this!

You can see up to 600 images a day all around you. Computers, TVs, billboards, and magazines display these images, which all send a message, but these messages aren't always true or helpful.

It's important to know which messages are useful and truthful and which ones are untrue or negative. Be cautious of negative messages that try to influence your thoughts or the way you feel about yourself. Nobody is perfect. Even actresses and models have photographers or a team of makeup artists and hairstylists to primp and polish them. This isn't what they look like naturally!

The more you accept and love your body, the more confident you'll feel. One way to start loving your body more is to remind yourself that you are beautiful and unique. Say it out loud, into the mirror!

FROM EMBARRASSED TO COMFORTABLE

Have you ever been embarrassed? I know I have! If you've ever noticed your face turn red or felt like you wanted to hide from everyone, that's embarrassment. It can be caused by anything that makes you feel silly or worry about what others think of you. Maybe you mispronounced a word while reading aloud in class, or you tripped and everyone saw. Embarrassment happens, and it's perfectly normal.

Embarrassment can stick with you and feel like it's never going to go away. It's important to know that it *will* go away, and you're not the only one feeling like this. Whenever you're feeling embarrassed, try to remember all the wonderful things that make you special. And remember, when a classmate does something embarrassing, you don't think about it all day, so they probably don't think about something you did, either!

Although it's not nice to laugh at others, it's definitely good to learn how to laugh at yourself. By learning to laugh at yourself with friends and family, you can turn embarrassment into confidence. Each time you feel embarrassed, think of it as a small step on a ladder toward self-confidence. As you learn to be comfortable laughing at yourself, trust that you're growing into the best person you want to be.

FROM SHY TO BRAVE

You might know a friend or a classmate who has always been very quiet. Maybe others call this person "snobby," "bratty," or "too quiet." But some people are just shy and keep to themselves—and that's totally okay. Shyness is a feeling of being uncomfort-able speaking up or talking in front of others. Kids who are shy feel more comfortable keeping quiet or staying in the background so that they aren't noticed or looked at.

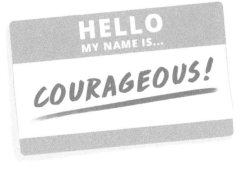

Sometimes shyness is a natural part of someone's personality, but sometimes it comes from a worry of not being accepted. If you've ever been the new kid at school, you know it can be hard to open up and begin making new friends. This is a good example of how being shy feels. Kids who feel shy want friends just like other kids do, but they feel less comfortable joining in.

Being shy can make someone feel lonelier than they want to. If you are shy, there are things you can do to give yourself the courage to speak up.

One way is to begin writing down things you can say in group settings or with a new friend. When a group of friends is doing an activity that you're interested in, you could say, "Hi, my name is _____! Mind if I join?"

Another good way to build courage is to ask another kid about themselves. This can be easier if they are a new kid or seem to be shy or alone also. You could ask them their name, their favorite sport, or how they did on the math test. With practice, you'll soon have the courage to ask if they want to hang out sometime!

Remember that being shy and keeping to yourself on the playground isn't the same as being careful around strangers. Only talk to adults who you know are trusted grown-ups. If you're scared to speak up in class or on the playground, then you might be experiencing shyness. If you're cautious around a stranger who is trying to talk to you, then you're being smart and safe.

FROM ANXIOUS TO CALM

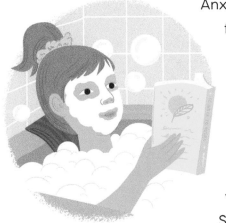

Anxiety is a feeling that comes from fear. Fear is a "primary" emotion we have, like sadness, happiness, and anger. Fear and anxiety can be helpful emotions. They can help keep us safe when our body and mind decide that we're in danger.

Sometimes our brain makes us think we're in danger even when we're not. It does this to help keep us safe, but too much of it can cause us to feel worried all the time. Too much worry can cause you to feel tired, and it can take up space in your mind that should hold fun, positive thoughts instead.

You may feel anxious around big dogs, before sports team tryouts, or when you walk into school. There are different types of anxiety, and all of them are normal every now and then. If you're scared of spiders, big dogs, or getting shots at the doctor, then you might have a phobia or fear of these things. If you feel anxious about leaving your mom or dad or staying the night at a friend's house, then you might have separation anxiety. If you're worried about a big exam or being liked by your friends, then you might be experiencing some general anxiety. These are all common. Usually, using the tricks we talked about on pages 13 to 21 will help, such as mindfulness, exercise, or self-care. While certain fears can be normal, they are no fun to live with every day. If any of these types of anxiety become too hard to deal with, tell a trusted grown-up or your school counselor.

FROM ANGRY TO PEACEFUL

Anger can be a tough emotion to deal with, because we don't feel totally ourselves when we're angry. Anger is only a feeling. It is not who we are. When we're angry, our brain is so busy trying to make sense of what we're angry about that it doesn't let us think straight. When we're able to think clearly, we make better decisions and we're usually kinder to others.

Has your brother or sister ever blamed you for something they did? Maybe you got even with them, and then you were the one who got into trouble. There are better ways to deal with anger. Counting to 10, going to your imaginary "safe space," or writing down what you want to say to them can all help you think clearly before acting.

Maybe when you're angry, you like to scream into a pillow or squeeze your fists into a tight ball. Maybe your friend likes to stay quiet and prefers no one talk to her until she feels better. No matter how you act, it is okay, as long as you aren't hurting anyone else or yourself.

Bullying

No one likes being bullied, and no one deserves it, either.

Bullying is a common but often painful issue that can cause deep feelings of anger, helplessness, and isolation. But bullying itself can sometimes be a result of anger, frustration, jealousy, or sadness. Have you felt any of these emotions and hurt a friend or sibling but then felt bad about it afterward? Not dealing with your feelings in a healthy way can sometimes lead to bullying, whether you mean it or not. Dealing with your emotions in a healthy way, like doing deep breathing or talking things out, can help keep you from hurting someone else whenever you're hurting.

There are different ways to tell if you're getting bullied. If someone constantly picks on you, makes you feel bad, or leaves you feeling scared or anxious or like you don't want to go to school, then you might be getting bullied. Bullying can happen in person as well as online.

continued >

If you think you're being bullied:

1. Tell a trusted grown-up or mentor right away. Tell more than one grown-up if you need to.
2. Do what you can to avoid the person who's bullying you.
3. Stick with a friend.
4. Tell the teacher if the bully is in your class.
5. Change up your body language to appear more confident. Practice your superhero pose in the mirror while saying phrases like "Leave me alone" in a strong and powerful voice. You can say it to the bully when you feel safe and ready.
6. Don't keep it inside! Talk about it with those you trust.

Additionally, if the bullying happens online:

1. Don't respond.
2. Save the post.
3. Share it with a trusted grown-up. Together, find out your school's policy on online bullying and report it if you can.
4. Make sure your settings are private and block that individual.
5. Leave the scene—take a break from social media for a while.

FROM SAD TO HOPEFUL

Sadness is another one of our "primary" emotions, like happiness and anger. Whenever our body and mind experience a "primary" emotion, we notice them quickly because they often feel a lot stronger than other emotions. Sadness is a tough feeling, but it's also a natural and healthy emotion to have every now and then.

There are many different reasons we may feel sad. We can't tell our brain when to feel sad or not feel sad—it just happens! But we can choose to deal with it in the best possible way. Things that help fight off sadness might include playing music; dancing; drawing; doing a favorite sport, activity, or hobby; talking to a good friend; or standing in front of a mirror and saying positive things.

Grief is a type of sadness that sits in your mind after you've experienced a loss, like when someone you loved has passed away. Maybe a relative or pet recently died, and you've noticed more feelings of sadness or even anger. Grief can feel really strong and make you want to cry. Other times, you'll be able to go about your day, laughing and playing with friends. Grief can stick around or come and go. It is just a strong type of sadness that reminds us of how special that person (or pet) was to us and how much we will always love and remember them.

To help yourself deal with these feelings, try drawing or painting your grief. What does it "look like" to you? Maybe it's a dark rain cloud or a big scribble with lots of dark colors. Maybe there are bright colors in there, too, as you think about that person. Talking about your feelings and noticing how your grief and sadness feel in your body can help, too. Maybe one day you want to cry and another day your stomach aches or you aren't hungry—these are all normal signs of grief and sadness. Whether it's from losing a loved one or dealing with a situation at school, sadness is an important feeling that we all have, and it's a healthy one. However, if you feel strong sadness every day for most of the day, it's a good idea to tell a trusted grown-up like your parent, school counselor, or family doctor.

FROM JEALOUS TO GRATEFUL

Has your sibling or friend ever received more attention than you? Maybe they won a contest, or did a solo in the concert, or scored the game-winning goal. Maybe they were sick and everyone was fussing over them. You may think they're more important than you in that moment. You may start to compare yourself to them.

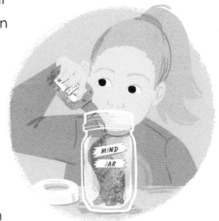

But comparing usually doesn't make anyone feel better; it only makes the feeling of jealousy stronger. You may even notice that you start to feel angry, or you try harder for your parents' or friends' attention. If your sibling is getting more attention from your parents, you may act out or misbehave to get some of their attention, too.

Jealousy is like pulling a dark curtain over your own special qualities, so you can't see them in the moment. When you're feeling this way, remind yourself what makes you special and unique. Do an activity that you know you're good at. While doing this activity, practice mindfulness and pay attention to your creativity.

You may notice that someone else is feeling jealous toward you and you don't know how to handle it, like a brother or sister during your birthday party. Maybe they don't understand why you're receiving special attention, and they're acting out. Remember to be kind and patient with them.

Feeling jealous does not make you a bad person. Ask yourself, "Why am I feeling like this, and what can I do to accept it and deal with it in a healthy way?" Maybe you can put yourself in the other person's shoes and consider how they would feel. How would you want to be treated if you were them?

Catch yourself if you start to compare yourself to others. You could say to yourself, "I think I'm feeling jealous. Let me think of things I am thankful for instead of things I am jealous of."

FEELING GRATEFUL

We all have things in our lives that make us happy, thankful, and grateful. But sometimes we can lose sight of what they are.

To practice gratitude, get a notebook or a few sheets of paper. Write the day of the week and something that makes you feel grateful today. This can be anything at all! If you're having trouble, try thinking about your day or looking around the room for things you're happy to see. This can be the macaroni and cheese on your lunch tray, the new friend next to you, your soccer ball, or the shoes on your feet.

Congratulations! You just started a gratitude journal. This helps you remember what's special and important in your life. You can write a grateful message daily and look at it when you're having a bad day. Just open your journal and remind yourself of all the things that make you feel your happiest.

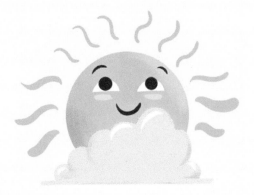

HELP ANDY FEEL BETTER

You've learned so much! Now choose the best advice to give your friend Andy, who might be experiencing similar feelings:

1. Andy is afraid of presenting in front of the class tomorrow. It makes her feel very nervous. You:

   a. Tell another friend and laugh together at Andy.
   b. Tell Andy you're nervous, too, and remind her that you will be there for her after the presentation to talk if she wants to.
   c. Make Andy feel silly for being nervous by saying, "Give me a break—you need to get a grip."

   Answer: B *Reminding Andy that she is not the only one who is feeling nervous is a good way to connect with your friend and remind each other that these emotions are perfectly normal. Offering support and a listening ear is a great way to be there for a friend, and it will show her that she can be there for you in this way one day, too.*

2. Andy keeps following you around at a party because she is feeling shy. You:

a. Try to shake her off by hiding in a bathroom.
b. Introduce Andy to people you know and tell them something they have in common, like, "Hey, aren't you both in the school choir?" Encourage her to join you in activities.
c. Tell Andy she needs to back off because it is annoying you.

Answer: B *Helping someone who is shy get out of their comfort zone is kind and a great way to build your own confidence. It's also fun to do this together, because you're making new friends and memories at the same time.*

3. You heard that Andy said something untrue about you to other friends. You:

a. Calmly ask her if she can talk later and set aside a time for you, her, and maybe even a trusted grown-up to talk out the problem. Maybe this is a misunderstanding or not even true.
b. Start saying mean things about her to your other friends.
c. Tell her you're no longer going to be friends.

Answer: A *Talking problems out is a helpful way to solve a problem without causing more problems in the meantime. If needed, a trusted grown-up can offer advice and keep the conversation from getting too mean or angry.*

4. A classmate is picking on Andy for being taller than the rest of the kids in the class. You:

   a. Join your classmate in making fun of Andy, because you did not like that Andy was taller than you.
   b. Tell her to pick on the classmate for being shorter than her.
   c. Suggest to Andy that she make a list of what she loves about herself. Remind her that everyone's body is different and she is beautiful just the way she is.

   Answer: C *Making a list of what she loves about herself will remind her what she's proud of and that everyone is unique and has awesome qualities. Your compliments will also help her feel good about herself.*

5. Andy comes to school angry because her parents made her apologize to her brother. She feels like she didn't do anything wrong. You:

a. Tell her, "Get over it. I just lost my homework."

b. Show her how to do deep breathing, and encourage her to wait until she is calm and ready to talk to her parents.

c. Tell her it's okay for her to be mad all day and treat others unkindly since she is angry.

Answer: B *You'll help Andy calm down by showing her deep breathing or whatever tricks work for you. This way, she won't hurt anyone else because of her anger, and she might have a better, happier day.*

6. Andy tells you she's been having negative thoughts all day and doesn't know how to stop. You:

a. Show her your trick for how to change a red thought to a green one (page 27) and see if she wants to practice it with you.

b. Tell her, "Don't worry. I'm sure they'll go away soon. It's no big deal."

c. Laugh at her negative thoughts when she shares them with you.

Answer: A *Now that you're a pro at turning red thoughts into green ones, show her your trick and let her know that it's totally normal to have red thoughts some days.*

7. Andy tells you that she thinks she's getting bullied on the playground, but she's not sure and is asking you for advice. You:

a. Ask her what the person is doing and suggest she talk to a trusted grown-up or teacher right away. Check in with her later and make sure she got the help she needed.
b. Tell her to confront the person on her own.
c. Laugh at her and say, "No one is a bully at our school. You'll be fine!"

Answer: A *By doing this, you're letting Andy know that you care about her safety, but you're also pointing her in the right direction to seek help from a trusted grown-up.*

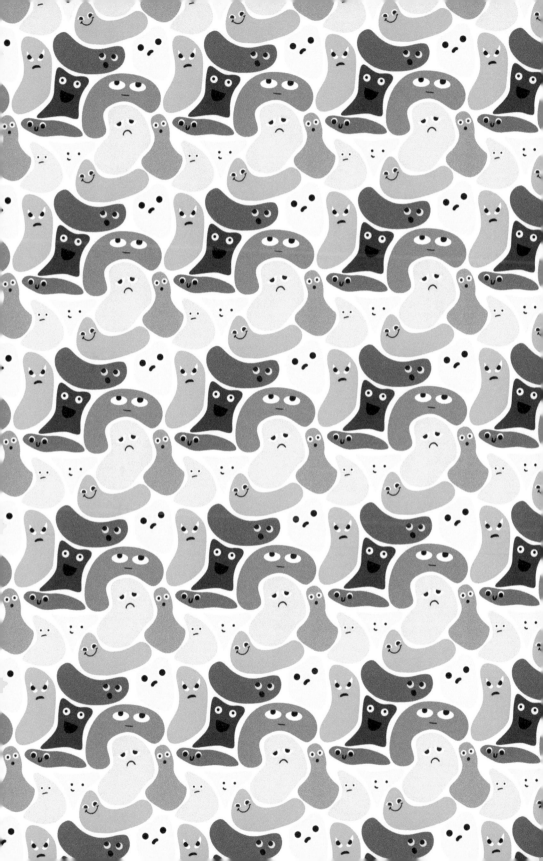

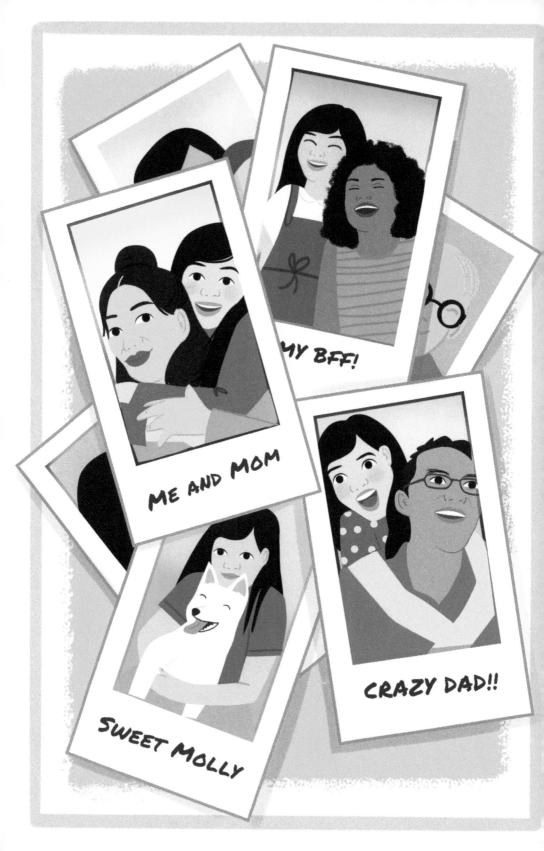

MY CHANGING RELATIONSHIPS

You are changing, and you may also be noticing changes in your relationships with others. You might feel more sensitive when your teacher corrects you in class, or more self-conscious around friends. These changes are perfectly normal! Whether they happen with your family, a friend, or a classmate, there are healthy ways to handle them.

We all like being with people who treat us kindly, laugh with us instead of at us, and listen when we need to talk. Friends are the people in your life who know what you're going through and accept you no matter how happy and silly you choose to be.

But as you grow, you may feel uncertain about these friendships. You might even notice some friendships will change—sometimes because of fights, peer pressure, or even just new interests. While it can feel sad or confusing to drift away from a friend, you are not alone—this happens to almost everyone! I'll share some good tips to help you work through these changes and even see the bright side of things.

You may start to notice changes taking place at home, too. Maybe when you were younger, you talked to your family about everything, but now you feel self-conscious when your parents ask you questions. Maybe you think they won't understand, or you just want your privacy. This is all a part of growing up.

It can help to look at these changes as the beginning of growth and strength within yourself. Let's talk about different ways to handle these changes so you can stay true to your wonderful, strong self and still feel connected to the people you love.

FRIENDS

There are times when a trusted grown-up is the best person to talk to. But friends can offer a different, special kind of support. Friends have a unique way of relating to you, laughing with you, and listening to you. Have you and a friend ever made up a language or secret hand-shake? That's a way of communicating that only you and your friend have. These types of friendships are important because they keep things fun and not-so-serious!

But along with friendships come some serious things, like peer pressure, making new friends, ending friendships, and dealing with bullying and cliques (a tight circle of friends). We all make new friends and end old friendships throughout our life, and that's normal. No one does this perfectly, but let's talk about some of the best ways to handle these issues.

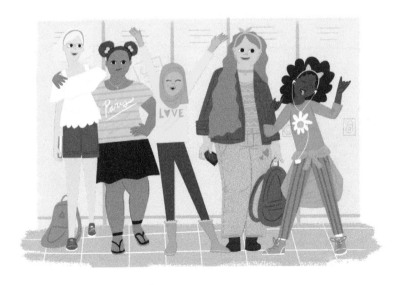

Making New Friends

Do you remember when you made your very first friend? You might not if you were very little. Humans have a natural ability to make friends even at a young age, because somehow, our body and mind know that healthy friendships keep us happy! There's always room for new friends, no matter how many you already have. But making friends can sometimes feel scary, right? You may worry that no one will accept you, or you might get frustrated when you feel left out.

Guess what? You already know some tricks to use to make yourself feel better when you're nervous about making new friends. Try changing up your body language, relaxing, or turning your negative thoughts into positive ones. You wouldn't want a negative thought to trick you out of becoming friends with your future best friend, would you? Remember, fear and worry can be helpful, but they can fool us sometimes.

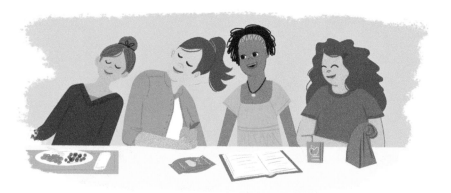

I trust that you're going to make new friends in no time, but here are a few tips to help you make those connections:

- ◆ Try to be kind.
- ◆ Show interest in others.
- ◆ Ask friends questions about themselves.
- ◆ Be a good listener.
- ◆ Give compliments.
- ◆ Make plans to hang out outside of school, not just in class.

If you feel nervous when trying these, that's a good sign. It means you are brave and growing.

Every day is a chance to make a new friend or learn from someone new. It might be hard to imagine right now, but you will have all kinds of friends come and go and some will be a better fit for you than others.

Making new friends doesn't mean you have to forget about your old friends, either. You can bring your old and new friends together by introducing them to one another to form one big, fun group. You could say to a new friend, "I have a friend that I've known for a few years. I think you'll like her, too. Do you want to meet her sometime?"

But don't settle for any friend, new or old, who has repeatedly hurt your feelings or isn't kind to you. Sometimes it's time to step away from a friendship if it doesn't feel good anymore. There's no need to fight or be unkind—just give the relationship a little space. Maybe it will work out and you'll be friends again, and maybe it won't, but it's important to choose to be around people who make you feel good about yourself and whom you can have fun with.

Cliques

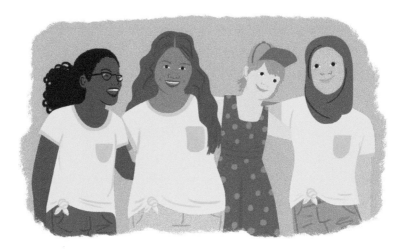

As you make new friends, you may notice you all grow into one big group of friends that do everything together. Or maybe you prefer to hang out with one or two of your closest friends in a smaller setting.

No matter what you prefer, you will likely be a part of a group at some point in life. There are many different types and sizes of groups out there. Small groups, large groups, sports groups, church groups, groups that do arts and crafts. You can start your own group and invite anyone who wants to join, like a dog-walking or scrap-booking group. Maybe even a group where you teach your dog how to scrapbook! Just kidding—that might be a little difficult.

There are all kinds of personalities in groups, but that's the wonderful part about them. In a good group, everyone is included and invited, no matter what.

Cliques are a little different. A clique is a tight group of friends. This might be a group of kids who all play basketball or musical instruments, but it may also be a group of kids who just enjoy each other's company. These groups can feel like "your people" and give you a feeling of belonging. A good clique will never try to change who you are, make you feel left out, or make you feel bad about yourself.

Some cliques are not so positive. A bad clique may gossip or make silly rules that try to control you. In a clique, you might only be allowed to wear blue or have to sit in the same spot every day at lunch. People in these cliques might not be "allowed" to talk or hang out with anyone outside of the clique, which isn't very fun or nice. You might notice more peer pressure in cliques or feel like you can't be yourself.

If you are feeling controlled, left out, or bullied by someone in a clique, step away and know that there are plenty of groups and friends out there who would love for you to join them. If you need help finding a group to join, start by telling a friend or trusted grown-up what you're interested in and see if they can suggest the right group for you.

No matter if you're a part of a group or clique, try to remember others' feelings and always be inviting. These experiences begin to shape the person you are going to be for life. As the saying goes, "Whatever you are, be a good one."

Peer Pressure

As you grow older, you'll learn more about what you like or don't like, who you are or aren't, and what you're comfortable with. Sometimes this will be fun and easy, and other times it can be hard and confusing. The important thing to know is that you don't have to let anyone pressure you into doing something that doesn't feel right.

It's easy to stick up for yourself around people you aren't worried about, like family and old friends. But what about the people in your life whom you like and want to be liked by in return—like peers, classmates, and new friends? When we're worried about being liked, it can feel harder to say no or be independent. Saying no and making your own decisions doesn't make you bad or boring. It makes you strong and a leader. You already have the strength within you to stay true to your values and awesomeness— so let's practice how to do it!

When you're feeling pressured or having a hard time deciding what to do, make three lists on a sheet of paper, colored red, yellow, and green (or pick your favorite colors).

Let's pretend Jamie wants you to help him pick on the new kid.

Your red list has reasons not to do something, or the reasons you're feeling uncertain.

Examples: I don't want to be mean to someone; that would hurt their feelings.

The yellow list has reasons you're thinking about doing something—are you feeling pressured, or do you think it would be fun?

Examples: I want Jamie to like me; I don't want to be picked on myself.

The green list, your "personal list," has your special qualities, or reasons you feel proud of yourself. (You could name this list "my special qualities" or decorate your name at the top.)

Examples: I always try to be kind to others; I do what I want, not what others tell me to do.

Think about all three lists or share the lists with a trusted grown-up who can help you decide. Is it more important to look cool to a classmate who is pressuring you? Or is it more important to stay true to who you are?

Consent

Your feelings and body are your own and no one else's, and you have the right to privacy and comfort. Just like you might need permission to use the Internet or walk to a friend's house, others need permission to touch or talk to you in a certain way. When you give permission, you're **giving** consent.

Getting consent means getting permission from others, while considering their feelings and respecting their privacy and comfort. Some people don't want to be hugged or talked to in a certain way, and that's okay.

Consent isn't just for in-person conversations. It's also for anything online. You're allowed to ask others to not talk to you a certain way online if it makes you uncomfortable, just like you're allowed to do in person. If you take a group photo with friends, it is important to remember that not everyone shares their photos, so you need to ask for consent before posting it online. And in return, nobody has the right to share your photo or information online without your consent.

If you're uncomfortable and do not want to be touched or talked to, you have the right to say, "Please don't touch me." This type of statement doesn't make you rude. It reminds others to respect you. Practice these statements with a friend or a trusted grown-up, or in the mirror by yourself, so you feel comfortable using them in public.

If anyone makes you feel bad for asking for consent, they're probably not someone you want to be spending time with. Most importantly, if someone does something without your consent, no matter how small or big, please tell a trusted grown-up. That's what trusted grown-ups are for.

Social Media

Social media can be exciting and dangerous all at the same time. Social media can make us feel happy and allow us to connect with our friends by messaging them or posting goofy photos together. Maybe those friends live in another state or country, so it can be extra special to connect with them.

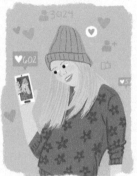

As fun and helpful as it can be, social media can also lead to drama, fights, or hurt feelings. If you see pictures of your friends doing fun things together, it can make you happy to see them, but it can also make you feel jealous or left out.

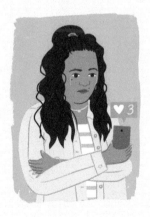

If you're noticing more negative feelings than positive ones, try taking a break from social media or ask your parents to help you spend less time on it. If you share your feelings about it with a trusted grown-up, they'll be able to help when you're feeling bad or unsafe when using it.

continued >

Also remember that anything you share on the Internet is always going to be out there. It doesn't go away, so you'll want to be careful and thoughtful about what you post or share with others.

It might feel cool or trendy to sign up for social media or download certain apps, but most social media platforms require you to be at least 13 years old before joining. These rules are designed to help keep you safe, happy, and healthy.

Here are few ways to make sure you're using social media safely:

♦ Make sure your profile is private so you can control who sees your posts.

♦ Ask a parent or trusted grown-up to help set your profile to private and block anyone who makes you feel uncomfortable.

♦ Never talk to strangers on the Internet, even if someone says they are a kid, looks like a real person, or says they know someone you know. A lot of people pretend on the Internet, and it can be hard to know who is telling the truth.

FAMILY

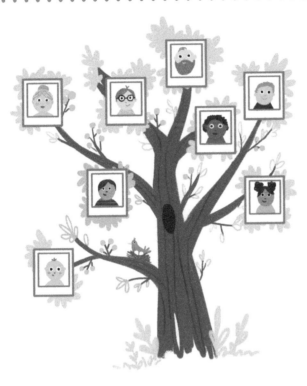

Families come in all shapes, sizes, and forms—big families, small families, families with stepparents, families with only a mom or dad, families with two moms or two dads, families formed by adoption, families who have experienced a loss, and many more. You may be close to your parents, or you may live with and be cared for by aunts, uncles, or grandparents. No matter the shape or form, your family's job is to support you, guide you, and stand by your side during whatever changes you're going through.

Roles and Responsibilities

Every family has its own pattern of relationships between family members and a different way that everyone acts around each other. This pattern will shift throughout life as you and your family members grow and change. Your mom or dad could be going through their own changes, like moving into a different house or getting a new job. Maybe you're the youngest in the family, and your siblings treat you like the "baby." As you grow older, you'll notice that you have more responsibilities, and you deserve to be treated like the young adult you're blossoming into. If a family member gets sick or has passed away, that can cause a shift, too. These shifts and changes can make your emotions feel stronger or harder to deal with.

Changes and shifts happen with every family. Treat your family members like co-captains of your boat and let them help you navigate the big and little waves.

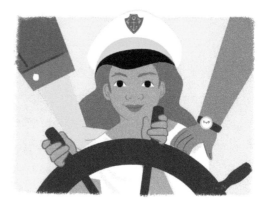

Getting Along

Maybe everyone in your family—dog, cat, and fish—are all getting along great right now. If so, hooray! That's great news. But maybe you and your sibling are fighting more than you used to, or maybe your feelings are stronger than before, and you don't think anyone would understand. Even if you're worried that your family members wouldn't get it, they do care, and it can be helpful to share your thoughts and feelings with them.

Activities, conversation starters, and games are some easy ways to break the ice so you can communicate with each other a little more easily.

A fun conversation starter is a question that starts with an introduction, like "When you were my age . . .?" Take it from here by asking:

- ◆ What was your favorite hobby?
- ◆ Who was your best friend?
- ◆ What subject were you terrible at?
- ◆ Do you remember having strong emotions as a kid? Did you understand them?
- ◆ Did you fight with your brothers?
- ◆ Were you ever embarrassed (scared, pressured, etc.)?
- ◆ What did you do for fun in the summer?
- ◆ What food did you like? What food did you hate?

This is a fun way to find out what your parents were like when they were your age. You may learn a lot about them and discover they aren't so different from you!

While games and activities like these are fun and can help you grow closer, you might feel like you need your own space, and that's okay, too. If you're feeling this way, you can use "I" statements (we'll talk about these soon) and ask for some personal space. You could say, "I am feeling anxious and would like some privacy to relax and do my deep breathing. Can I please excuse myself?"

Boundaries

As you grow, it's natural to want more privacy or boundaries. Boundaries are all about respecting one another's privacy. You might want to run into your sister's room and borrow her favorite dress, but as she gets older, she asks you to please knock first. (She may not always say it this nicely, but she is asking you to respect her boundaries.)

This works both ways, and you have boundaries that others should respect, too. Wanting more privacy or having more boundaries doesn't mean you're rude or want to spend less time with someone. Your parents and older siblings were your age once, too, and they know how important boundaries are.

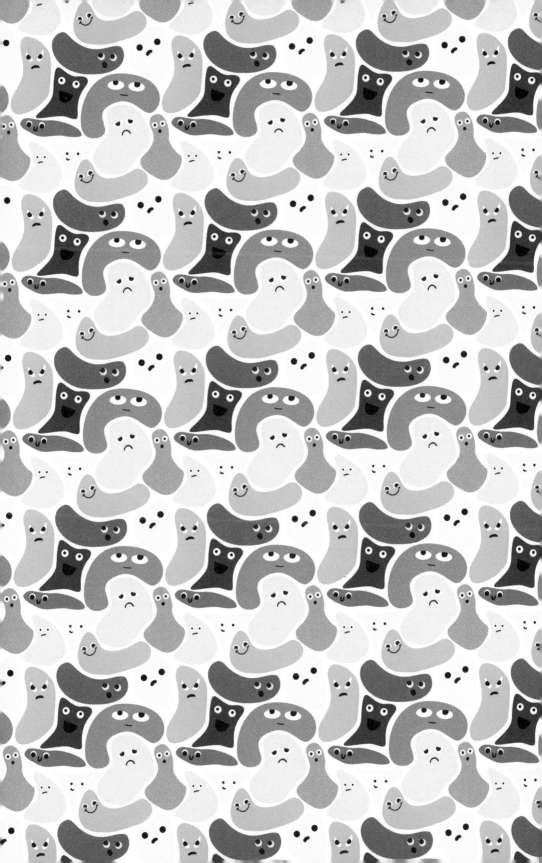

"I" STATEMENTS

"I" statements are honest messages that tell how you feel about something. They can help you say what you need and let others understand what you are feeling. And they all start with—you guessed it—"I." Here are some useful examples of "I" statements:

- ♦ "I feel anxious when you rush me in the mornings before school. Can we talk about things to do the night before so we aren't as rushed in the morning?"
- ♦ "I get mad when you don't look like you're listening. It hurts my feelings and makes me feel silly for talking. Would you please look at me?"
- ♦ "I feel embarrassed when you walk into my room. Can you please respect my privacy and knock first?"

Try it for yourself:

1. I feel _____

   when you _____

   _____

   _____

2. I feel _____

   when you _____

   _____

   _____

3. I feel _____

   when you _____

   _____

   _____

Asking for privacy, attention, and other things you need doesn't make you rude. It shows your maturity and growth. (You can even show your family this exercise so they understand where you're coming from!)

Love Yourself

It's normal to have all kinds of feelings at home, because we're usually more comfortable there than anywhere else. When we're comfortable, we tend to show our emotions a bit more. At home, you might feel anger, frustration, jealousy, and silliness all in one day. When you do:

◆ Remember that everyone has emotions, including everyone in your family. The important thing is that everyone respects feelings and each other and tries to listen.

◆ Find a safe place to try your helpful tricks, like mindfulness (page 18) or muscle relaxation (page 14).

◆ Talk it out with a trusted grown-up or friend.

◆ Write a list of what makes you special, unique, and strong.

◆ Express your feelings and get creative by drawing a family photo. If you're feeling mad at your family, draw your pets or friends instead.

ROLE MODELS AND MENTORS

Mentors are all around you. Think about your librarian, older sister, coach, or teacher. Many of these people act as mentors in your life simply by being themselves. Maybe your mentor is one of your family members or a friend's mom or dad. A mentor can be a parent figure, but they don't always have to be. Mentors want to see you grow and succeed, and they often listen well, give good advice, respect your boundaries, and have qualities you look up to. Think about the people in your life who care about you,

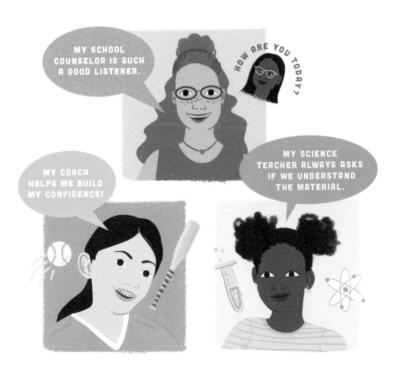

make things fun, and help you when you need it. If you want to learn more from that person, you can ask them if they can be your mentor. You could say, "I notice you help me with a lot, and I like learning from you. Could you act as my mentor?"

A positive role model is also someone you look up to and want to be more like. Positive role models have personality traits and qualities that you admire or that match up with your values or beliefs. Some of these qualities may be more obvious, like if they're smart or kind to others. Some may be less obvious, like if they're hard-working or humble. Unlike a mentor, a role model might not know you look up to them, because they could be a famous athlete, scientist, author, or politician whom you haven't met in person.

If you think you've found a positive role model or mentor, ask yourself what you like about them and make a list of the ways you want to be like them.

MY ROLE MODELS

Many qualities can make someone an awesome role model! Think about the people you admire and consider role models. Circle the qualities that describe them:

Kind	Knowledgeable	Brave
Positive	Funny	Accepting of others
Determined to do the right thing	Creative	Joyful
Honest	Determined	Emotionally strong
Not afraid to be themselves	Fun-loving	Caring toward others
Confident	A good communicator	A good listener
Understanding	Respectful	Humble

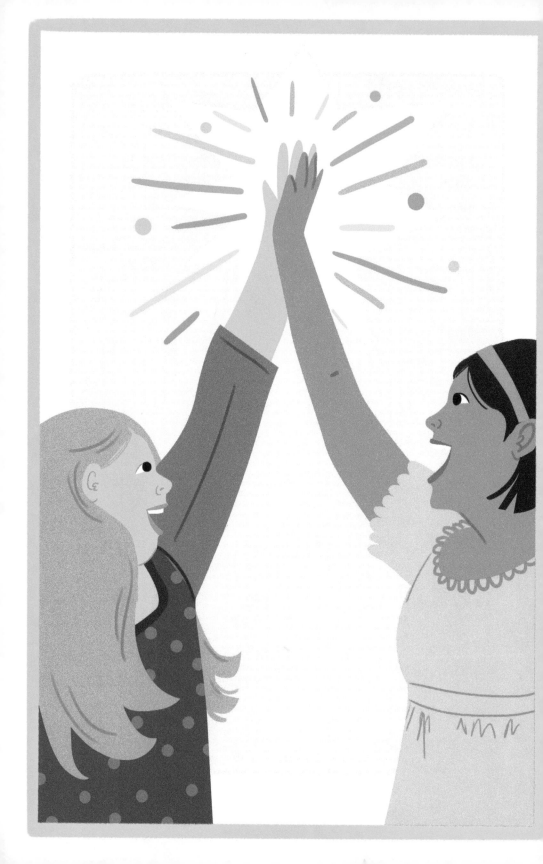

MY BEST SELF

. . . .

Impressed with yourself yet? I am! You've done some extraordinary work to get here. You've learned about the connection between your body and mind, your hormones, feelings, emotions, and changing relationships. You've learned great tricks for handling your emotions and completed all kinds of quizzes and activities along the way. Give yourself a high-five and think about everything you've learned—you are clearly in charge of your boat and its course toward a promising future! I hope you feel empowered, fabulous, and proud of the strong, confident person you are.

FEELING EMPOWERED

Have you ever been to a buffet where you could pile all the pizza and dessert on your plate that you want, but you knew this decision wouldn't be the healthiest? So instead, you grabbed some veggies or a salad for a healthier balance. As you grow, you'll be faced with a buffet of choices in life, and you'll have the power and responsibility to select the healthiest choices for yourself. Your healthy choices might look different from a friend's or sibling's, and that doesn't mean yours or theirs are wrong. You can be different and healthy at the same time!

With your new knowledge and skills, you have the choice to make good decisions and take care of yourself and those you care about. Let's talk about some of the skills you've learned that you can choose to use:

- ✦ You can manage strong emotions in ways that work best for you.
- ✦ You can think more positively by turning red thoughts into green ones.
- ✦ You can use good body language to feel and look more confident.
- ✦ You can be kind toward others, and you can love and care for yourself.
- ✦ You can help your friends learn the skills you have for managing strong emotions.

- You can accept ups and downs with friends and understand that your friends are going to go through their own changes, too.
- You can take steps to make new friends or identify and leave an unhealthy friendship.
- You can choose friends, groups, and cliques that work for you.
- You can respond to peer pressure and stay true to who you are and what you believe in.
- You can tell what makes a trusted grown-up and how they can help.
- You can use "I" statements to ask for what you want.
- You can set boundaries for yourself at home, in social situations, and online.

Knowledge is power, and you've got a lot to help you and to share with others. How empowering!

FEELING FABULOUS

Part of being human means you'll feel uncertain through-out life, and you may continue to wonder who you are as you grow up. We all wonder! The beautiful thing about life is that it is always changing and giving us the chance to be the best version of ourselves with each new day. Remember that your sister, brother, friend, classmates—even parents—are going through their own changes, and sometimes the way people feel or act has nothing to do with you or your relationship with them.

Remember, these changes and strong emotions aren't as powerful as your strength and confidence. Everything you're feeling is normal, and we've learned that there are healthy and unhealthy ways of managing it all. Using your favorite tricks to manage emotions is the best way to grow up great, like talking it out when you get into a fight with a friend or reminding yourself to take a few deep breaths when you're mad.

You might run into different kinds of situations not mentioned in this book that cause you to feel worried, jealous, excited, or disappointed. Trust that no matter what happens, you can count on yourself and your favorite tricks to get you through it and keep a positive mindset. You're one fabulous person, and I am so very proud of you!

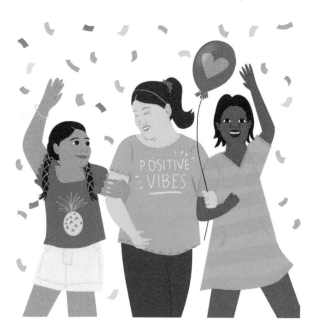

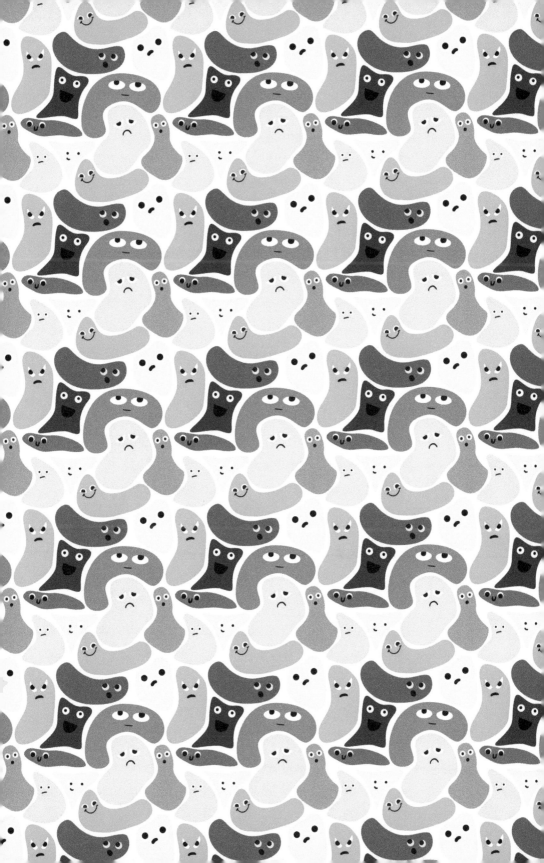

I FEEL...

· ·

Congratulations! You've finished this book and learned so many wonderful things about yourself and your changing emotions as you grow. I hope you feel as proud of yourself as I do of you.

Take a moment to think about your emotions and circle any feelings you have now that you've finished the book:

EXCITED	CAPABLE
UNCERTAIN	SAD
POSITIVE	FEARFUL
HAPPY	JOYFUL
CURIOUS	CONFIDENT
SILLY	EMBARRASSED
BORED	ANXIOUS
THOUGHTFUL	CHEERFUL

PROUD   GRATEFUL

HOPEFUL   COMFORTABLE

MAD   FRUSTRATED

STRONG   NERVOUS

CALM   EMPOWERED

SURPRISED   WORRIED

OPTIMISTIC   SAFE

SHY   SERIOUS

Think of your own and add them here:

_____

_____

Remember, you can always come back to this book to keep what you've learned fresh. The more you use these tips and tricks, the better you will start to feel.

RESOURCES

Here are some resources for you and your parents or other trusted adults to explore together to learn more about emotions, puberty, and just growing up great!

Print Books

Girls in Real Life Situations: Group Counseling Activities for Enhancing Social and Emotional Development, by Julia V. Taylor and Shannon Trice-Black

This book has so many great activities to promote social skills. It can be used both inside and outside the classroom and is easy to understand.

The Self-Compassion Workbook for Teens, by Karen Bluth, PhD

This workbook helps you progress in loving yourself in fun, interactive ways on every page. It's a book you can write in and use every day to remember to be kind to yourself, ignore your negative thoughts, and feel proud of who you are.

Being Me: A Kid's Guide to Boosting Confidence and Self-Esteem, by Wendy L. Moss, PhD

There are so many wonderful and relatable examples of self-esteem and self-confidence in this book that are sure to help any child, confident or not. This book offers tools for dealing with low self-esteem and helps children grow this confidence in any circumstance.

Online Resources

Always remember to ask for permission before using the Internet or downloading any apps.

Your Life Your Voice

yourlifeyourvoice.org

A great place to find everything you need in a crisis or when you feel like you have no one to talk to. It has numbers for hotlines or text lines, a Q&A section, and a "Tips & Tools" section.

GirlsHealth.Gov

girlshealth.gov

This site lets you explore everything in your life from friendship drama to the proper nutrition you should be getting, and even things that aren't talked about as often, like illnesses and disabilities, or environmental stuff like how to help take care of the planet.

A Mighty Girl

amightygirl.com

Find tons of age-appropriate recommendations for books, TV, movies, toys, and clothing. The website describes itself as "the world's largest collection of books, toys, and movies for smart, confident, and courageous girls." It sounds like a pretty awesome place!

Amy Poehler's Smart Girls YouTube Channel

youtube.com/user/smartgirls

This channel is designed for curious, smart girls like you. It has videos about everything from "modern texting manners" and making math fun, to interviews with amazing women like famous astronaut Dr. Jeanette Epps. The channel is catered a bit more toward older girls, so be sure to ask for permission before watching.

REFERENCES

MY CHANGING EMOTIONS

American Psychological Association. "Stress Effects on the Body." Accessed February 23, 2020. apa.org /helpcenter/stress-body.

Bailey, Regina. "The Limbic System of the Brain: The Amygdala, Hypothalamus, and Thalamus." *ThoughtCo.* Last modified March 28, 2018. thoughtco .com/limbic-system-anatomy-373200.

Bergland, Christopher. "Mindfulness Made Simple." *Psychology Today.* March 31, 2013. psychologytoday.com/us/blog/the-athletes -way/201303/mindfulness-made-simple.

Brain Made Simple. "Hypothalamus." Last modified November 13, 2019. brainmadesimple.com /hypothalamus.

BrightFocus Foundation. "Brain Anatomy and Limbic System." Last modified July 21, 2019. brightfocus .org/alzheimers/infographic/brain-anatomy -and-limbic-system.

Cherry, Kendra. "The 6 Types of Basic Emotions and Their Effect on Human Behavior." *Verywell Mind.* Last modified January 13, 2020. verywellmind.com /an-overview-of-the-types-of-emotions-4163976.

CHOC Children's Hospital. "Sleep Hygiene for Children." Accessed February 23, 2020. choc.org/wp
/wp-content/uploads/2016/04/Sleep-Hygiene
-Children-Handout.pdf.

Dusenbery, Maya. "How Exercise Affects 2 Important
'Happy' Chemicals in Your Brain." *Livestrong.com.* Last
modified October 18, 2019. livestrong.com/article/25
1785-exercise-and-its-effects-on-serotonin-dopamine
-levels.

Halloran, Janine. "Deep Breathing Exercises for
Kids." *Coping Skills for Kids.* Accessed February 23,
2020. copingskillsforkids.com/deep-breathing
-exercises-for-kids.

Healthy Brains. "6 Pillars of Brain Health." Accessed
February 23, 2020. healthybrains.org/pillar-physical.

Immordino-Yang, Mary Helen, and Vanessa Singh.
"Hippocampal Contributions to the Processing of Social
Emotions." *Human Brain Mapping* 34, no. 4 (October
2011): 945–55. doi.org/10.1002/hbm.21485.

Komninos, Andreas. "Our Three Brains—The Emotional Brain." *Interaction Design Foundation.* 2018.
interaction-design.org/literature/article/our-three
-brains-the-emotional-brain.

Lenzen, Manuela. "Feeling Our Emotions." *Scientific
American.* April 1, 2005. scientificamerican.com
/article/feeling-our-emotions.

MacMillan, Amanda. "Sleep Tips for Kids of All Ages." *WebMD*. November 23, 2015. webmd.com /parenting/raising-fit-kids/recharge/features /kids-sleep-tips#1.

Moawad, Heidi. "How the Brain Processes Emotions." *Neurology Times*. June 5, 2017. neurologytimes.com /blog/how-brain-processes-emotions.

Pillay, Srini. "How Simply Moving Benefits Your Mental Health." *Harvard Health Blog*. March 28, 2016. health .harvard.edu/blog/how-simply-moving-benefits -your-mental-health-201603289350.

Ramanathan, Mangalam. "Hormones and Chemicals Linked with Our Emotion." *Amrita Vishwa Vidyapeetham*. October 15, 2018. amrita.edu/news /hormones-and-chemicals-linked-our-emotion.

Thomas, David. "Don't Let Your Hippocampus Stop You from Being a Successful Investor." *Forbes Magazine*. May 10, 2018. forbes.com/sites /greatspeculations/2018/05/10/dont-let-your -hippocampus-stop-you-from-being-a-successful -investor/#3faff97d2694.

Young Diggers. "The Fight or Flight Response: Our Body's Response to Stress." February 2010. youngdiggers.com.au/fight-or-flight.

MY CHANGING MIND

Blakemore, Sarah-Jayne, Stephanie Burnett, and Ronald E. Dahl. "The Role of Puberty in the Developing Adolescent Brain." *Human Brain Mapping* 31, no. 6 (June 2010): 926–33. doi.org/10.1002/hbm .21052.

Coltrera, Francesca. "Anxiety in Children." *Harvard Health Blog*. August 14, 2018. health.harvard.edu /blog/anxiety-in-children-2018081414532#.

Ehmke, Rachel. "Helping Children Deal with Grief." *Child Mind Institute*. Accessed February 29, 2020. childmind.org/article/helping-children -deal-grief.

Hawkins, Nicole. "Battling Our Bodies: Under-standing and Overcoming Negative Body Images." *Center for Change*. Last modified August 2014. centerforchange.com/battling-bodies-understanding -overcoming-negative-body-images.

Jacobson, Rae. "How to Help Kids Deal with Embarrassment." *Child Mind Institute*. Accessed February 28, 2020. childmind.org/article/help -kids-deal-embarrassment.

KidCentral TN. "Social and Emotional Development: Ages 8-10." Accessed February 27, 2020. kidcentraltn .com/development/8-10-years/social-and-emotional -development-ages-8-10.html.

Rochat, Philippe. "Five Levels of Self-Awareness as They Unfold Early in Life." *Consciousness and Cognition* 12, no. 4 (December 2003): 717-31. doi.org/10.1016 /S1053-8100(03)00081-3.

MY CHANGING RELATIONSHIPS

Brotherson, Sean, Divya Saxena, and Geoffrey Zehnacker. "Talking to Children About Peer Pressure." *North Dakota State University*. October 2017. ag.ndsu.edu/publications/kids-family/talking -to-children-about-peer-pressure#section-3.

GirlsHealth.gov. "Friendships." Last modified November 2, 2015. girlshealth.gov/relationships /friendships.

Kennedy-Moore, Eileen. "Children's Growing Friendships." *Psychology Today*. February 26, 2012. psychologytoday.com/us/blog/growing-friendships /201202/childrens-growing-friendships.

MediaSmarts. "Internet Safety Tips by Age: 8-10." January 19, 2017. mediasmarts.ca/tipsheet/internet -safety-tips-age-8-10.

Smith, Leonie. "8 Year Olds On Social Media—What Parents Should Know." *The Cyber Safety Lady*. October 25, 2018. thecybersafetylady.com.au/2018/10/8-year -olds-on-social-media-what-parents-should-know.

Society for Adolescent Health and Medicine. "Mental Health Resources for Adolescents and Young Adults. Accessed March 8, 2020. adolescenthealth.org /Resources/Clinical-Care-Resources/Mental-Health /Mental-Health-Resources-For-Adolesc.aspx.

INDEX

ACKNOWLEDGMENTS

Researching this book has been both refreshing and humbling. I learned a thing or two about myself in the process and feel thankful to have been given this opportunity. This would not have been possible without those in my life who have pushed me out of my comfort zone toward the tough but necessary self-reflection required for this exciting book. Additionally, I am thankful for my dog, Goose, who is always by my side.

Last but certainly not least, thank you to all the young girls I've had the pleasure of working with and learning from. You've taught me so much about the beautiful journey you are on, and it has been a privilege to witness. You are all an inspiration to me and to each other, and I hope you see that.

ABOUT THE AUTHOR

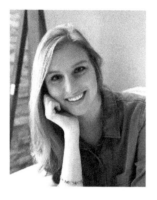

LAUREN RIVERS is a resident clinical mental health counselor specializing in child and adolescent mental health. Lauren works at a private practice clinic that specializes in play, art, and sand-tray therapy, and she is trained in eye movement desensitization and reprocessing (EMDR) and neurofeedback training. Lauren received her master's from Johns Hopkins University and worked in outpatient settings throughout the city and county of Baltimore.

In addition, Lauren is vice president of a nonprofit organization, Wings of Joanne, that provides respite care and entertainment to bedridden pediatric patients and their families through virtual reality and gaming consoles. Lauren knows the importance of the psychosocial well-being of these children and their families and presented on this topic at Princeton University in 2019.

She resides in Northern Virginia and enjoys exploring the greater DC area, but frequently takes trips home to spend time with her family on the beaches of Alabama and Florida. You can learn more about her interests and passions at LaurenRiversTherapy.com and WingsOfJoanne.com.